Intermittent Fasting 101

Powerful Intermittent Fasting Strategies To Burn Fat, Lose Weight and Build Muscle

Faith Evans

About The Author

Faith Evans is a mother, a wife and an entrepreneur. She has been following intermittent fasting from 2016 and has lost over 20 pounds. She writes books to share her experience with intermittent fasting, what has worked for her, what has not and how to be successful with losing weight with intermittent fasting.

against the publisher for any reparation, damages, or monetary loss due to the information herein, either directly or indirectly.

Respective authors own all copyrights not held by the publisher.

The information herein is offered for informational purposes solely, and is universal as so. The presentation of the information is without contract or any type of guarantee assurance.

The trademarks that are used are without any consent, and the publication of the trademark is without permission or backing by the trademark owner. All trademarks and brands within this book are for clarifying purposes only and are the owned by the owners themselves, not affiliated with this document.

Table of Contents

Introduction

Losing weight can be an uphill task. This is why various diets have come up to make the process a bit easier. Unfortunately, they fail to achieve their work simply because they are not practical.

Some diets often require you to restrict your intake of certain foods completely, which can intensify cravings while others need you to take questionable 'slimming pills' all in the name of losing weight. The downside of most of these very restrictive diets is that once you achieve your weight loss goal, and are done with the diet, you gain all that weight back and start the cycle again.

This does not have to be the case with you. There is a way to safely lose weight like I did, and still enjoy the foods you love and this is by adopting intermittent fasting. This book has all the information you need about intermittent fasting to lose weight and build muscle.

Chapter 1: How Intermittent Fasting Works

Intermittent fasting (IF) is not a diet. Rather, it is a pattern of eating. This is because it stipulates when you eat and not what you eat. With intermittent fasting, you have an eating window and a fasting period that allows you to take full advantage of the two states your body can be in.

What are these states? Well, these are:

The Fed State

One of the states your body can be in is the fed state. As the name suggests, this state is where the actual feeding, absorbing and digesting takes place. Whenever you take a bite to eat, you enter the fed state, and your body starts digesting and absorbing the food you give it. Your cells 'feed' on this food as it were.

During the fed state, one thing that will go up is your insulin production. Insulin is that hormone that helps your body to not only use but also store glucose. It is responsible for delivering the glucose right from your bloodstream into the muscles, fat and liver. As such, when insulin production increases, your body will cease burning fat and will rely on the glucose you give it.

The fed state typically lasts for 3-5 hours once you start eating. If you make the habit of eating after every 3-5 hours, your body will have plenty of food to use. It will also have plenty of excess carbs to store and this will lead to weight gain. As such, you must give your body the break it needs in between feedings to use up the energy already in your fat stores. This is where the fasted state comes in.

The Fasted State

If your body is not in the fed state, then it is in the fasted state. However, before you can fully enter the fasted state, your body has to go through a stage known as the post-absorptive stage. This stage typically starts 3-5 hours after you take your last meal. At this time, all the food you had eaten would have been absorbed into your bloodstream.

But there's something you need to note.

The post-absorptive stage can last 8-12 hours. During this time, your body will have access to the components of your last meal and the stored glycogen. Remember, carbs are converted to glucose so that the glucose can be used for energy.

Any excess carbs are converted to glycogen and stored in your muscles and live, and if any more carbs remain, they are then converted to fat and stored in your fat stores. Thus, in the absence of glucose, your body will start using its glycogen stores. Once the 12 hours are up, you'll fully enter into the fasted state. During this time, your body will be in need of refueling.

Here's the important part.

If you consume food just as you enter the fasted state, your body will again have access to all the glucose (energy) it needs. However, if you fast during this time, your body will have to adjust and use other sources of energy.

It will start by using up the glycogen stored in your muscles and liver. Once it is done, your body will turn to burning up the fat in your fat stores for its energy needs. When you are in this state, insulin levels decrease dramatically and this leads to fat burning. But that's not all. Your nervous system also does the job of sending a neurotransmitter and hormone known as norepinephrine to your fat cells. This facilitates the breakdown of your body's fat. Your body ends up with free fatty acids and these are effectively burned for energy leading to more weight loss.

But there's another hormone that is also affected during the fasted state.

This is the human growth hormone (HGH). This hormone is the one responsible for aiding fat loss and gaining muscle. During the fasted state, levels of HGH skyrocket. As such, your body will not only lose fat but it will be in a great position to gain muscle especially if you engage in fasted training.

Nevertheless, before you lose weight and gain muscle, you must give your body enough time to do so. This is why intermittent fasting protocols typically have at least a 16-hour fasting period. This is enough time to get into the fasted state and start burning up fat.

One of the most amazing things about intermittent fasting is that there exist different types of intermittent fasting and you can choose what suits you best. If you don't find something that you like, you can as well come up with a suitable method for yourself putting in mind the two body states and how to ensure you enter the fasted state.

The following chapter will look at some intermittent fasting methods and how to choose one that suits you best.

Chapter 2: Choose Your Fasting Protocol

The first step in achieving success with intermittent fasting is to choose an intermittent fasting protocol that will suit you well. This means taking your time and being honest with yourself in order to determine your pattern of eating and ways to change it to burn fat and build muscle. There are various IF protocols you can try out. These include:

The 16/8 Fast

The 16/8 Fast or Lean Gains as it is commonly called is an intermittent fasting protocol that was specifically designed to not only help people become 'lean' but to also enable then to 'gain' muscle, hence the name. This type of intermittent fasting method was popularized by Martin Berkhan and it has become the go-to fasting protocol for those who want to experience the benefits of fasting but don't want to wait for long hours before their next eating window.

When you start the 16/8 fast, you will have a 16-hour fasting period. This means that you're not allowed to consume calories for 16 hours. The fasting period is followed by an 8-hour eating window. This means that you can eat your food within this 8-hour window. Please note that you will not be eating continuously for eight hours. Rather, you can choose to have 2-3 meals during this time. As such, you have to state clearly, when you will start the fast.

For example, your fasting period can start at 10:00p.m at night and last up to 2:00p.m the following day. This will give you 16 hours to go without food. This means your eating window will be from 2:00p.m to 10:00p.m. This will give you 8 hours within which to eat your meals. The idea is to find an ideal time to start your fast and stick to it.

But, there's more.

When following the Lean Gains method, you are expected to stay active during your fasting period. This means no more sitting about waiting for the hours to pass by. You need to keep moving. You can engage in a variety of physical activities such as taking walks, doing house chores, dancing, working out etc. The idea is to give your body a good workout in order to burn more fat and build muscle.

Eat Stop Eat

Eat Stop Eat is an intermittent fasting protocol attributed to Brad Pilon. According to Pilon, the purpose of this protocol is to give yourself, a 24-hour break from eating. You can decide to engage in this type of fast once or twice a week. If you fast once a week, you will have 6 days to eat 'normally' and if you fast twice a week, you will eat normally for 5 days. The idea is to spend the whole 24 hours without consuming any calories during your fast days. However, you can still drink non-caloric drinks such as unsweetened coffee and water.

But caution is advised.

Here is the thing. It is not easy to stay without eating for 24 hours especially if you are used to eating several meals in a day. This means you will need to find ways to combat temptation. The best thing to do is to remain busy as you go about your day. Always remember your goals. The fact that you will only be fasting once or twice a week should encourage you to stick to intermittent fasting.

But there's something else you need to keep in mind.

Fasting for 24 hours is not an excuse to go overeat once you break your fast. As has been said, you will be eating normally for 5-6 days. These are many days compared to your fasting period. Thus, if you overindulge during your normal days, you will sabotage your weight loss efforts and that won't do you any good. Therefore, it would be prudent to keep an eye on what you eat and try to stick to the amount of calories you should eat for the day. This is normally 1600 calories for women and 2000 calories for men.

The Warrior Diet

The warrior diet is a fasting protocol that involves a 4-hour eating window followed by a 20-hour feeding period. It is modeled after warriors of old. In the past, warriors tended to stay busy throughout the day and did not have the chance to eat a full meal until late in the evening. Of course, they could nibble on things like fruits and nuts they found along the way but often times; they only had one big meal at the end of the day.

With this protocol, you stay without eating any food for 20 hours. However, you can snack on fruits or raw veggies. If you decide to eat snacks, you must remember that snacks also contain calories and that calories add up at the end of the day. Your goal is to burn fat and the only way to achieve this is by limiting the amount of carbs you consume. But as you'll find out, once you get over the initial hunger pangs, your body will get the energy it needs from fat burning and your hunger pangs will cease.

However, you need to prepare yourself to consume a huge meal once you break your fast. Remember, you will only have a 4-hour eating window. You have to consume all your calories within these 4 hours. Take your time to enjoy your meal and snacks during this eating window.

It is usually advisable to start with protein and vegetables when you break your fast, and only eat carbohydrates when you feel that you are not satisfied.

The 5/2 Diet

The 5:2 diet is an intermittent fasting protocol that allows you to eat as normal for 5 days per week. It also stipulates that you fast on 2 nonconsecutive days. During these fasting days, you can eat up to 600 calories if you are a man and up to 500 calories if you are a woman. The food you eat can be distributed throughout the day as long as you stick to eating the amount of calories allowed. As such, you can choose to eat a single meal, two meals or even three meals on the fasting day. However, if you choose to distribute your calories, you will have to be very careful to add them up so as not to overeat.

The 5:2 diet can help you lose weight but it is also useful as a maintenance diet. This means that you can use other fasting protocols in order to lose a significant amount of weight before using the 5:2 diet to keep your weight in check.

Remember that you still need to avoid overeating during the days you are not fasting. Remember, excess carbs will be stored in your body. If you overeat 5 days in a week, you will be sabotaging yourself. However, if you eat the amount of calories you need, you will be providing your body with the right tools it needs to lose weight and keep the weight off.

Once you determine your fasting protocol, put it in writing. State clearly what time you will be in the fasting period and what time your eating window will be. You should start your fasting period at the same time each day to make it easier to track your progress.

Chapter 3: Ease Into Intermittent Fasting

As much as you would want to jump right in and embrace intermittent fasting, this is not advisable. Remember, you will be changing your pattern of eating. This is not something you should do lightly or abruptly. Changes come with their own challenges and thus, it would be best to make them slowly.

The idea is to slowly increase the number of hours you stay without food until you arrive at the number of hours you would want to be in the fasting period. If you do this, you will have enough time to adjust and this will go a long way in guaranteeing your success. The changes you need to make include:

Don't snack after dinner

As has been said before, when you consume food, your body is said to be in the fed state. This means that it is constantly using up the food you are giving it. Thus, it does not have the chance to use up the food in its stores. If you wish to lose weight, it is only prudent that you strive to get into the fasted state where your body can put your food stores to good use.

The first step in doing this is by avoiding late night snacking. Don't eat anything that contains calories until the next day breakfast. If you have to, put your kitchen under lock and key until the morning.

Delay breakfast

Once you do away with late night snacks, you can take another step. You can gradually delay the time you take your breakfast. For example, if you usually take your breakfast at 7:00a.m, you can now take it at 8:00a.m, which may mean changing your morning routine. If the first thing you do after you wake up is grab a bite to eat, you want to create a new habit. In this case, you may want to read the paper or check your mail. But whatever you do, don't consume calories. If you wish to consume unsweetened coffee and other non-caloric beverages, go ahead. That would be acceptable.

Skip breakfast

Many people find it easier to skip breakfast rather than trying to skip dinner. This is because there is usually a lot going on during the morning hours. This is the time you plan for your day and ensure you have all you need to make your day successful. You'll probably be running up and down as it is. Thus, you won't miss not eating your breakfast once you get used to the idea of not eating it. Remember, you will already have delayed your breakfast by some hours. Thus, it will reach a point where skipping it altogether will make more sense to you especially since you will want to get into the fasted state so that you can start achieving your goals.

Eat your dinner early

Apart from skipping breakfast, you can also have your dinner early. As always, keep in mind that you need to be in the fasting period in order for fat burning to take place. If you have decided to opt for a 16-hour fast, you'll only have an 8-hour eating window but this will be followed by a 16-hour fasting period. If you have your dinner early, you won't have to wait very long to break your fast once you wake up. This will make IF more appealing. For example, if you have your dinner at 6.00p.m, you will be able to have another meal as early as 10.00a.m.

But overall, you need to make intermittent fasting work for you. The strategies you employ should make your life easier and not harder. Of course, you will need time to adjust but it should not be a struggle. Intermittent fasting should mesh into your lifestyle. Even as you lengthen your fasting period, there is one thing that can help you navigate it successfully. This is redefining your hunger.

Let us learn more about this in the next chapter.

Chapter 4: Redefine Hunger

Hunger is one thing that can derail your weight loss efforts. When you are hungry, you are tempted to reach out for whatever food that is nearby in order to satisfy that hunger. Unfortunately, if this occurs during your fasting period, you will interfere with fat burning.

So, what can you do?

You can redefine hunger. This simply means looking into the type of hunger you are feeling and finding ways to hold off from eating so as not to mess up your fasting period. Types of hunger include:

- Mind hunger – This is the type of hunger that you feel when you know it is time to eat'. Many people are brought up knowing that certain times mean mealtime. Thus, when the clock strikes, their mind shifts to food even when they are not hungry. Remember, you do not have to eat just because the clock says it is time to eat.

- Mouth hunger – This type of hunger arises when you see something or smell it. For example, you catch a glimpse of a tasty cake and your mouth begins to water as if you can already taste it and suddenly, you want it. This is why you need to remove temptation. Lock away your food until it is time to eat and do not stare at food you are not supposed to eat. It will do you no good.

- Teeth hunger – This type of hunger is usually brought on by anxiety or irritation. It makes you want to chew away your frustration in a not so gentle manner. You are not eating because you are hungry but rather, you are using food as a punching bag. As such, you would do better to find healthier ways to deal with frustration.

- Thirst – Thirst is often confused for hunger. When you are thirsty, your body needs water not food. Unfortunately, the signal it sends resembles those of physical hunger. As such, you find yourself reaching for food. Instead of doing this, drink some water the next time you feel hungry.

- Fatigue – When you are tired, you may find yourself eating something in order to 'replenish your energy'. This should not be the case. You need to rest if you are feeling tired, not eat.

- Emotional hunger – This type of hunger is brought on by the difficulties of life. You may have heard of emotional eating. Some people turn to food when they are feeling sad or depressed. However, you also need to watch out when you are feeling happy. It's not unusual for people to celebrate milestones or good news with food. That still falls under emotional eating. Learn to find ways to express yourself without turning to food.

- Physical hunger – This is the type of hunger that causes your stomach to rumble. It signals that your body is in need of refueling.

While there are various types of huger, one thing they have in common is that they all signal your body to reach out for food. While physical hunger is said to be the 'real' hunger, you cannot ignore the signals other types of hunger present. However, you can learn to recognize the type of hunger you are dealing with and this will help you to quickly deal with the root cause of the hunger instead of reaching for food.

But what if you are confronted with physical hunger? Should you break your fast? No.

Think about it. What is the purpose of eating food? You eat food to refuel your body and get the energy you need to live and carry out various activities. The keyword is energy. Your body is signaling you to consume food because it needs energy. The good news is that your body can get the energy it needs from various sources. It does not have to rely on glucose. In fact, if you don't feed during your fasting period, you will give your body an opportunity to tap into your glycogen and fat stores.

What does this mean for you?

It means you can afford to stay without food and allow your body to burn fat. Yes, you may feel hunger pangs especially during the first few days of IF. However, such hunger pangs will lessen if you do not eat. You have to stay strong and keep in mind how IF works and the reasons you are doing it in the first place. This will motivate you to wait until your eating window before you consume any calories. The good news is that once your body adjusts, you'll find it easier to stick to your fasting period. A great way of making it through your fasting period is taking some drinks. The following chapter will provide you with some drinks that you can take.

Chapter 5: Staying Hydrated

The truth is that many people don't take in as much fluids as their body requires and those who do, normally do so during mealtimes. Thus, when fasting is added to the mix, there is a real danger of dehydration if you don't take precaution.

The good news though is that you can consume several drinks during your eating window and fasting period. Such drinks come in handy when you have to abstain from eating. First, they keep your body hydrated and secondly, they help keep hunger at bay by keeping your stomach full. However, the best part is that they will not stop your body from burning fat. That is a major win.

Some drinks you can consume during the fasting period include:

Tea

Tea is something that many people enjoy. You don't have to stop drinking tea during the fasting period. Tea reduces your hunger pangs and it is quite useful when it comes to reducing abdominal fat and LDL cholesterol. It also contains a good amount of antioxidants that help in the fight against disease. Green tea is especially recommended for weight loss. However, there's a catch. When you drink your tea, you are not supposed to add any cream or sugar. You have to drink it as it is. Some people add sweeteners, which is okay as long as such sweeteners don't contain calories.

Coffee

Coffee is one beverage that many people enjoy especially before they start their day. You can drink it several times during your fasting period. However, it is advisable you do not reach for it immediately you wake up. This is especially so if you still have some hours to go before you break your fast. You can use a cup of coffee to get your mind of hunger but you need to monitor your intake.

Yes, coffee is good for your metabolism and it has disease-fighting antioxidants but it also tends to cause some irritation to some people. If you find yourself becoming irritable, experiencing an upset stomach or having an increased heart rate just because you've drank coffee, then it is time to rethink your drinking habits.

The goal is to make fasting easier, not to add health issues to your life. Don't add any milk or sugar to your coffee if you do decide to drink it although you can add cinnamon and such like spices if you wish.

Water

Despite various blogs and articles talking about the importance of drinking water, people don't just drink as much as they should. By the time, your body complains that it needs water, you may drink one or two glasses and that is it. That is far from the 8 glasses experts say you need to drink.

Water is great especially during your fasting period because it keeps you full. It also does a good job of flushing out toxins that you may have as your body breaks down the fat for energy.

If you just don't like the taste of water, you can add some lemon slices to make it a little bit more palatable. Remember not to get carried away and start chewing the fruits or putting too much of them in your water. You are trying to make it a little bit more palatable, not trying to create appetizing cocktails. It should still be recognizable and it should not keep you from burning fat.

Apple Cider Vinegar

Apple cider vinegar is a beverage often associated with intermittent fasting due to the benefits it brings. It has been shown to improve digestion and regulate blood sugar. Apple cider vinegar works to enhance the effects of fasting. You can take 2-3 tablespoons of this beverage per day.

Broth

Broth is not something you should drink during most fasting protocols. However, if you are doing a 24-hour fast, then you will benefit from taking vegetable or meat broth. The idea is to get the nutrients in the broth and remain hydrated throughout the fasting period. As such, leave out the meaty chunks or the juicy vegetables. You will basically be drinking the 'soup' not eating the solid pieces.

Of great importance with intermittent fasting is ensuring that you do not overindulge in food because this will negate all the benefits you gained. In addition, it is advisable to opt for healthy foods. While intermittent fasting is not to strict in terms of the food you can eat during the eating window, eating healthy and nutritious food is great for you.

The following chapter will focus on cleaning up your diet so that you eat the right nutritious foods during your eating window.

Chapter 6: Clean Up Your Diet

The main reason people gain weight is that they consume more food than their bodies need especially excess carbohydrates. Processed food, refined sugar and junk food largely contribute to this. They are not only more palatable but also easier to digest. They also contribute to something known as carb addiction. This is where your body craves more and more carbs simply because eating carbs makes you feel good. It gives you a kind of high that is comforting. However, once that high elapses, you are left feeling sluggish as you experience a carb crush. Unfortunately, many people react to this by eating more food and this just leads to more weight gain. This is why you need to clean up your diet.

What does this entail?

Clean eating simply means eating the type of foods that are better for your health. It means minimizing the amount of processed food and refined sugars you eat. Rather than eating processed food, you get to eat food in its natural form or as close to it as possible.

Let us learn how you can ease into clean eating since as with anything, starting something new can be challenging:

Load up on fruits and vegetables

Fruits and vegetables often make an appearance whenever people try to lose weight. This is because they are loaded with vitamins, minerals, and fiber while being quite low in calories. They also not only keep you full but help protect your cells and fight inflammation.

One way to increase your consumption of fruits and vegetables is to eat them in salads. When you make your salad, you should try to make it as colorful as you can, using a variety of vegetables and greens. You can add things like apples, oranges or berries to your salad. You can also toss your salads with olive oil and herbs. The good thing about salads is that they can serve as a full meal and you can have them as a snack when you want to eat something light before your main meal.

You can also make it a point to substitute vegetables in various recipes. For example, if a recipe calls for rice, you can use cauliflower in its place. This way, you will minimize your intake of refined carbs and increase your consumption of vegetables.

Limit processed food

Highly processed foods and refined carbs should not feature in your day-to-day diet. This is because such foods have been modified into something that is different from their natural state. They have added chemicals and toxins that should not be put in your body, and they are highly addictive since processing makes them more palatable and easier to digest. Thus, you will not only eat more of such foods but you will want to eat them often. In other words, when you eat highly processed foods, you will increase your chances of gaining weight.

Instead of eating highly processed foods, you should endeavor to eat whole foods. Whole foods contain more nutrients and fiber and they promote gut health and reduce inflammation. Make small but significant changes to your diet and you won't be disappointed. It may take some time to get used to the 'new' taste, but your body will adjust and thank you for it.

Limit sugar

Sugar is sweet. It makes your food tasty. Unfortunately, it adds little nutritional value to your life but, it does add on the calories. If you are trying to lose weight, you have to greatly limit added sugars and stop using high-fructose syrup. The thing about added sugar is that it appears in many foods. You can find it in foods like sauces, condiments, cookies, breads and so forth. Since it makes food sweeter, you will find yourself eating more of such foods and this will contribute to weight gain.

If you have to use sugar, you should try out natural sugars such as honey and maple syrup but remember that natural sugars should also be limited. If you consume them at every meal, you will add on the pounds.

Avoid packaged snacks

When you are trying to lose weight, one of the things you should avoid is packaged snacks such as Potato chips. Snacks give your mouth something to chew on and most of them tend to contain sugar, salt and trans fat. These things will not help you. Another thing about snacks is that in most cases you cannot just seem to get enough of them. Once you open that package, you will find yourself dipping your finger into it every now and then until the snack is all gone.

If you want to eat snacks, you should oft for healthy snacks such as fruits or healthy, homemade snacks such as kale chips. You can also snack on a handful of nuts. The idea is to eat something small during your eating window in between main meals. But don't forget to count the calories you get from snacks. They too will contribute to the overall calories you consume.

Avoid vegetable oils

Vegetable oils and spreads happen to be highly processed and they are linked to weight gain, inflammation and heart disease. Additionally, most of them contain the dreaded trans fats that is just not good for your health. This is why you need to avoid vegetable oils.

Vegetable oils are usually be found in fried foods and other processed food. If you eat such foods, you will not only sabotage your weight loss efforts but also put yourself at a risk of suffering from certain diseases. Instead of consuming vegetable fats and spreads, opt for healthy oils and fats such as olive oil and coconut oil.

Eat organic

As much as possible, you need to shop and eat organic. Factory farms are good at mass-producing food and animal products. They usually use chemicals and hormones to maximize growth. Animals, especially, are kept in closed spaces. Such places are a recipe for disease outbreak. In order to prevent the spread of disease, factory farms give the animals antibiotics and this affects the quality of the meat.

What's more, most factory farms give the animals grain to feed on instead of things like grass that animals such as cattle naturally feed on. As such, the meat produced is of poor quality.

So, what can you do?

Well, you need to be more conscious when shopping for your food. It is not enough to buy the food and hope for the best. You need to do some research and find out what type of food you are actually buying. Organic products are usually labeled as such. It is up to you to know where to find them and take the step to choose organic whenever you can. This way, you will be consuming healthier foods.

Cleaning up your diet has benefits now and in the future. If you clean up your diet, you will be able to lose more weight now and you will increase the chances of keeping that weight off in the future. However, there's something else you can do to lose weight and gain muscle. This is fasted training. Lets see what this is about.

Chapter 7: Engage In Fasted Training

Fasted training simply means engaging in various exercises during your fasting period. There are good reasons why you should engage in fasted training. The first reason is that fasted training helps you burn more fat. Remember we talked about your body using its glycogen stores before turning to fat burning. Well, training on 'an empty stomach' speeds things along. It ensures that your body taps into those storehouses.

However, there is another good reason you should engage in fasted training.

Fasted training takes advantage of the human growth hormone. As we saw earlier, the levels of HGH increase when you are in the fasted state. This increase is said to go up to a 5-fold increase. Thus, engaging in fasted training will enable you to make good use of this muscle-building hormone.

In order to embrace fasted training, you should:

Determine your workout routine

Yes, you can work out when you are in the fasted state but you have to be smart about it. This is especially so if you are used to sitting down the whole day. You have to start slow and allow your body to get stronger before you increase the intensity of your workouts.

There are basically two types of workouts you can engage in during your fasted state. These are cardio workouts and anaerobic workouts. Let us look at each of them.

Cardio

Short cardio sessions (less than 50 minutes) are suited for fasted training. This is because they will help you to increase your aerobic fitness. Cardio-based workouts are geared towards helping you lose weight and increase your endurance rather than focus on muscle gain. Athletes are attracted to such training sessions because fasted cardio helps increase VO2 Max, which is the amount of oxygen you can consume when you are doing an aerobic workout. If you effectively improve your ability to take in oxygen, this will enable you to work harder as your muscles will have all the oxygen you need. Thus, if you are a runner, you will greatly benefit from this type of workout.

However, if you want to build muscle, you are better off with doing short bursts (20-30 minutes) of anaerobic exercises such as weight lifting. A good workout routine to engage in is the Big 3.

The Big 3

The big 3 training routine consists of the squat, deadlift and bench and it is designed to get you strong and ripped. You can do it 3 times a week with a rest day in between workouts. For example, you can workout on Monday, Wednesday and Friday. The routine is recommended for beginners and it can be done at your own pace.

When you're doing this routine, you use a fixed rep system. This means that you should use the same weight for all your workouts. It is also advisable for you to consume 10g BCCAs before your workout and then consume 10g BCCAs in 2-hour intervals until you break your fast. This will help build your muscles and aide in recovery as you workout.

The idea of the workout is to finish one exercise and then move to the next and then the final exercise before resting for 30-90 seconds. Once the resting period is over, you move to the next rep. For example, you can do 5 squats, 5 deadlift and 5 bench press. That will be one rep; aim to do 5 reps. Also, determine how long you'll be resting for in between reps and use a stop watch to keep your rest time the same.

When you are doing the big 3, the idea is to start lifting the weight you are comfortable with and then gradually increase that weight as your form improves. As such, you will still be doing the same amount of reps but with a heavier weight. When you are comfortable with the exercises, you can add another rep and more weight. Many people add 10lb weight for the squat and deadlift and a 5lb weight for the bench press. Over time, you will find it easier to lift more weight but if you're struggling to do the exercises, there is no harm in reducing the weight until you're more comfortable.

Stick to the plan when doing your workout routine. Remember that everyone started from somewhere. Do not try looking cool and taking on too much. You will achieve your goal as long as you work at it diligently. Once you're done with your workout, you need to break your fast.

Consume your post-workout meal

After your workout, you need to refuel your muscles. This will help with regenerating and recovery. You should aim at refueling within 20-30 minutes. Some of the foods you can consume within 20-30 minutes post-workout include:

- Muesli and fruit

- Banana and oats

- Omelet and rye toast

- Eggs, toast, avocado and veggies

As a rule of thumb, you should aim at consuming at least half of your calories for the day once you are through with your workout. You can consume a whole-food meal and follow it up with a high-calorie shake.

If you're doing a 16-hour fast, your schedule should look something like:

- 10 AM – Fasted state strength training.

- 11 AM – Break your fast with a whole food meal and a high-calorie shake. This should constitute half of your calories.

- 6 PM – Eat your remaining calories.

- 7 PM-11 AM – Enter a 16-hour fasting period.

You can plan to train earlier or later but endeavor to follow a similar schedule. The idea is to do your workout just before you break your fast. You want to build muscles, not break them down. The food you eat just after your workout is integral to recovery and regenerating. Plan accordingly and while you're at it, figure out ways to avoid stress because stress can make it difficult to stick to intermittent fasting and even lose weight.

Chapter 8: Manage Stress

Stress is something your body goes through in response to anything it thinks can attack it; hence, stress is normal though it can get out of hand. When you are stressed, your body responds by releasing a hormone known as adrenaline. This 'fight' or 'flight' hormone prepares your body to deal with a stressful situation.

Adrenaline comes with a rush of energy and a racing heart among other symptoms. It prepares your body for physical action and it is very helpful when you are in danger and you need to take quick action. However, if your body is in a continuous "flight" or "flight" mode, then there is a problem. It will mean dealing with various symptoms of stress that will no doubt put a toll on your body.

Symptoms of stress include:

- Racing heart

- General aches and pains

- Trembling/shaking

- Dizziness

- Grinding teeth, clenched jaw

- Increase in or loss of appetite

- Headaches

- Cold and sweaty palms

- Indigestion or acid reflux symptoms

- Upset stomach, diarrhea

- Tiredness, exhaustion

- Muscle tension in neck, face or shoulders.

- Sexual difficulties

- Problems sleeping

- Weight gain or loss

As you can see, such symptoms are not desirable. They wreck havoc in your body and the do not give you any time to rest and rejuvenate. Over time, these symptoms will interfere with your life.

But, why do you need to get rid of stress?

Well, as we've seen, stress comes with a variety of symptoms that can interfere with your day to day life. In light of what we are discussing, it is important to note that one of the symptoms of stress is weight gain.

When you are stressed, you may find yourself turning to food in order to seek comfort. It is common to hear people talking of 'comfort food'. Comfort food simply means the food you turn to when you are feeling low, stressed or depressed. It is usually high in carbs. This is because carbohydrates make you feel good since they work on your brain's pleasure center and bring you 'comfort', which therein lies the problem

Before long, you'll want to eat such food again. You will become a 'couch potato' as you continuously munch on junk food as you try to 'eat the blues away'. In the end, you'll just add on to your problems as you gain weight and put yourself at a higher risk of suffering from stress-related health issues. This is why it is important to learn to manage stress. Below is a variety of techniques that you can use:

Write it down

A good way to deal with stress is by writing about the things that stress you. You can start by describing the situation and your feelings towards it. Note down the things such as the person involved, what was said and how you reacted to it. Later, look at your notes and then determine how you could have dealt with the situation and use the lessons you learn to deal with similar situations.

Another thing you can do is imagine various scenarios and ways to deal with them. This will prepare you to face similar situations in future.

Laugh

Laughter is good for relieving stress and getting your mind off your problems. However, you should not wait until you are sad to look for something to lift your mood. It is important to figure out things that make you happy so that you can include them in your life.

For example, things such as funny videos, cartoons and comedies can make you laugh. You can use them as a form of release. You can also find happiness in developing a skill, playing a game or even cooking. The idea is to find a project and celebrate every milestone you achieve as you try to complete it. Once you complete the project, you will bask in the happiness that comes with doing a job well and this will lift your mood.

Laughter is important because it shows you that there are many things to celebrate in life. Life is not just about your challenges and struggles. It is also about your accomplishments and the little things that bring you joy.

Master your time

The way you use your time will affect your stress levels. If you do not manage it well, you will constantly find yourself rushing to accomplish things. This will keep your stress levels high and you will not be able to react to situations in the best way or make informed decisions. Your life will be about reacting to one issue after another instead of planning and determining what you want to spend your time on.

You can easily change this if you take the time to list down the things that you need to do and determining their level of importance. The idea is to finish the urgent and important tasks first before you can spend your time on other things. This way, you will always have enough time to do high value tasks that affect your life.

Learn to say 'no'

It is important to note that you have the right to say 'no' when you are not in the best position to carry out requests. If someone wants you to do something, it is up to you to gauge the situation and determine whether you can fulfill the request without harming yourself.

Doing something requires you to use your time and energy. They take a piece of you and such; you need to be careful where you spend your energy. If you spend it on things that only drain you, you will not have enough energy to spend on things that are important to you.

Use essential oils

Essential oils and scented candles are often used to soothe away anxiety and improve sleep. You can use scents such as lavender, roman chamomile, bergamot and ylang ylang.

The trick is to breathe in the scents as you go about your day. You can use a diffuser to diffuse essential oils into the air you breathe or you can carry a bottle of your favorite oil and use it when you are feeling stressed.

Overall, you need to keep in mind that the things you are dealing with will affect your health and your diet. If you have healthy ways to deal with issues, they will not overwhelm you and this will make your life easier.

As you adopt intermittent fasting, you will need to learn more about being mindful and in the moment. Let us learn why this is so important:

Chapter 9: Practice Mindfulness

Mindfulness is all about being in the present instead of constantly living in the past or thinking about the future. It is about dealing with things as they occur and paying attention to what you are doing in the moment.

Mindfulness is important as it helps you appreciate the things you have in life. When you are mindful, you learn to take a moment to enjoy what you are experiencing and this greatly improves the quality of your life.

When you practice mindfulness, you will be less prone to succumb to stress. Instead of worrying about things that happened or imagining the worst-case scenarios, you will have the opportunity to appreciate the little things that show you there is a lot to celebrate in life even if you are going through tough times. Thus, things like stress eating will not be an issue for you. Let us learn more about mindful eating

In order to embrace mindful eating, you should:

Eat first, then shop

There is something about shopping while you are hungry that makes you pick up things you would not pick up if you were full. When you are hungry and you see food, you want to eat as soon as possible. This means buying things such as ready-made processed food that you can eat on your way home. It also means buying more of certain foods that you know can easily fill you up. This is why you should never shop while you are hungry. Instead, eat first and make a shopping list based on your needs instead of on the things you want.

Read labels

When you shop, you need to develop the habit of reading labels. Labels tend to list the ingredients contained in food products. You want to watch out for ingredients that have names that are difficult to pronounce. Foods that have added sugars and chemicals should not feature in your diet.

Another thing you need to do as you determine what foods you will eat is take a moment to think about the process that the food went through to reach you. Think about the farmers, the planting and harvesting process and the journey the food traveled before it reaches you. This will give you greater appreciation of the food you eat. It will also help you make better choices when selecting food.

Be present during food preparation

Food preparation is one activity you can find joy in if you allow yourself to embrace it. Instead of going about it subconsciously, you need to put more effort into what you are doing. For example, you can pay attention to the way you wash your vegetables, the sound of the knife as it hits the board, the sound of your blender as it pulses food and so on. If you have kids, you can use this time as a teaching opportunity. Children who are picky eaters will normally try things they have made. This can be a way to teach them about food and expand their food options.

Just eat

Once upon a time, families made it a point to sit at the tables for their meals. They would eat as they chat about their day. This practice does not occur as often nowadays. Nowadays, things such as phones, TV, social media and computers are often present during meals. People eat as they continue to work or chat on their phones. As a result, they eat at a faster pace and do not pay attention to what they are eating. Before they know it, what they were eating is finished nd they have no idea how that happened or even how much they ate.

Food is meant to be enjoyed. If you are to do this, you need to pay attention to each bite you take. This means removing distractions and sitting down at the table for meals. It also means taking time to chew your food before you even think of the next bite.

Don't ignore your fullness cues

When you are eating, there reaches a time when you begin to feel full. You need to stop eating at this time. This is because your stomach takes a few minutes to catch up to your brain's fullness cues. By the time you start to feel full, you are well on your way to overeating. Mindful eating brings attention to your fullness cues and allows you to stop eating knowing that your body already has what it needs in terms of calories.

Mindful eating changes the way you interact with your food. It makes you more conscious about the choices you make and this will work well to help you make better choices when you're on IF and long after you stop practicing intermittent fasting. Let us now look at your perception of intermittent fasting and how it can definitely affect your weight loss journey.

Chapter 10: Change Your Perception

Whenever people hear the word 'fasting', they often picture going for days without food and all the negative connotations that accompanies the word fasting. If you are used to eating 3-6 meals a day, the idea of going without food for an extended period can seem like a punishment.

This is not what intermittent fasting is about.

Rather, intermittent fasting is about affording you more freedom. It gives you the freedom to spend less money on food as you will be eating fewer meals. You will also spend less time on meal planning, food preparation and cooking. As such, you need to view intermittent fasting as the good thing it really is. Its purpose is to enable you lose fat and gain muscle. It will make you feel good, look good, have a sharper mind and feel more energized. Those are desirable benefits indeed!

But as we've said, it may be challenging to get a proper view of fasting. But you can do a number of things to help you with that:

Normalize IF

When people go on a diet, one of the first things they are advised to do is tell someone about it. They are advised to tell their family members, friends and colleagues about their diet. This is said to create accountability and motivate the person to stick to the diet.

As we have already seen, IF is not a diet but rather a pattern of eating. Rarely do we let everyone know when we decide to eat something unless we are planning to invite them to share in the meal. Thus, it is not necessary that you tell people that you are planning to fast.

Think about it. A diet is supposed to be done within a certain period. It is supposed to show results within that time. On the other hand, intermittent fasting can be done for a prolonged period. Some people embrace it fully and don't even think about it as it becomes their new normal. There is an advantage to this. Sticking to intermittent fasting will ensure you do not put back the weight you have lost even if you do indulge in your favorite foods from time to time. Your body will still have time to tap into its fat stores. However that is not the main reason you should normalize IF.

Normalizing IF, stops you from being overly concerned about what you are eating. For example, if you time the 16/8 fast such that you break your fast at 10:00a.m that will seem as a small thing once you get used to it. You will just know that you eat breakfast at ten and dinner at 6:00p.m and that will become your new normal. Thus, you won't think of fasting as this thing that requires you to put in a lot of effort. Rather, you will think of it as something reachable you excel at each day.

Stay busy

You need to stop thinking of fasting as something that will cause you to look malnourished and lose energy. That is definitely not what intermittent fasting does. Yes, there are people who fast for prolonged periods due to religious and political reasons. You are not those people. You are fasting in order to lose weight and build muscle. That is why you want to engage in intermittent fasting not long fasts. You will likely be fasting for less than 24 hours. Thus, there is no need to develop a 'woe-is-me' attitude. You are not starving. Your body still has access to the energy it needs to function properly. So, don't spend all day sleeping or sitting around lamenting how hungry you are as you eagerly await your next meal. You need to be busy and keep moving.

Don't get carried away when breaking the fast

One thing you need to keep in mind is that breaking a fast is not an opportunity to overeat. You were not starving. You do not need to bulk up on food in anticipation of when next you will not be eating.

Intermittent fasting is a conscious decision to stop eating for several hours. You are still in control and your food will be waiting for you once it is time to eat. Thus, instead of reaching out for that junk food you have been craving, break your fast with something light. Eat things like soup, fruit and vegetables. These foods will be easier on your stomach as you break the fast. You can eat a heavier meal later if you want to but once again, don't overdo it.

Don't be fooled by labels

Human beings like labeling things. Unfortunately, labels tend to mislead more than they help. Someone picks up something labeled 'low-fat' thinking it is better than the regular stuff because of what is associated with the label. They do not stop to think of the processing the product has gone through and the additions it has to make it that way. That is what labels do; they give you a false sense of health.

You may have heard of things such as healthy eating or something already discussed here, clean eating. These are labels, and they bring with them a list of foods that are healthier for you. However, what you need to understand is that too much of a good thing is also bad for you. If you overeat healthy foods, you will add on the calories and sabotage your weight loss goals. You have to be practical. You can do this by keeping an eye on your calories.

Think energy, not food

There is a big difference between needing food and needing energy or calories. Food satisfies physical hunger. It gives as the calories we need. However, as we have seen, your body does not have to use up whatever you eat at that moment. It can use up whatever you have stored.

As such, the next time you're feeling hungry, don't think of food. Think of energy. Tell yourself that your body needs energy and that it knows where to find it even if you eat nothing. If you do this, you will wait for your body to kick-start fat burning instead of reaching for food. This will allow you to stick to your fasting period.

Conclusion

We have come to the end of the book. Thank you for reading and congratulations for reading until the end.

As you have learned, intermittent fasting can be a powerful tool when it comes to losing weight and building muscle; but, you need to do it right. Once you choose an intermittent fasting protocol that suits you, start slow, watch what you eat and change your perception, you will be well on your way to losing weight. In addition, if you engage in fasted training, you will increase your chances of building muscles. So, what are you waiting for? Try out Intermittent Fasting today, lose the weight, build muscle and enjoy all the other amazing benefits intermittent fasting has to offer.

Finally, I would like to ask you for a favor. Can you please leave a review for this book? I will greatly appreciate that.

Thank you and Good Luck!

Thank You

www.ingramcontent.com/pod-product-compliance
Lightning Source LLC
Chambersburg PA
CBHW051417250726
48655CB00003B/1104